DEREK PANELL

How I Lost Over 21 Pounds in 30 Days

My Daily Journey to How I Lost over 21 Pounds in 30 Days

This book was professionally typeset on Reedsy.
Find out more at reedsy.com

Contents

1 Introduction   1

2 Support System   3

3 What to Expect   4

4 Shopping List for Version from Health Advisor   6

5 The Daily Plan Version 1   7

6 My Shopping List   9

7 My Daily Plan for 30 days   11

8 Why I had to Change Up My Plan   13

9 Exercise   15

10 Water   19

11 After the 30 days   21

12 Conclusion   23

1

Introduction

I ntroduction

Welcome to my Journey of My Weight loss to lose over 21 pounds in 30 Days. My name is Derek l and I'm extremely excited to share with you this step by step process.

I will tell you what I ate, drank and did personally for a month to lose this weight. I'll make it as simple as possible to help you along the way.

My whole life I have been struggling with my weight from fad diets to magic pills and starving myself. I know I had to change what was going on. I was over 400 pounds, Yes 400 pounds. I was always active but would be tired and need a nap. I take walks and many trips to Florida to see friends. Days by the pools walking around to the restaurants and shops and the theme parks. I would walk 10-15 miles a day without thinking and I see the numbers and say wow that's crazy. The toughest thing was for me when I went to the Theme Parks in Florida and couldn't ride certain rides due to my size. Yes I was very embarrassed but felt left out and had to wait for my friends to go on rides and roller coasters as I watched. I have spent thousands of dollars through the years with limited results or regaining the weight back rapidly.

Also I personally didn't have any medical issues such as diabetes, sugar, high blood pressure and didn't wanna have any of that. So I needed to change for Me and for my Quality of life.

2

Support System

S **upport System**
Everyone needs help. Find a friend or family member to help and support you. I Lucky have a Great group of friends that support and check in with me. I get Calls and texts from a buddy Andrew in Florida. Shout out to the Florida and Califorina Friend network. Lyle, Divina, Chris, Jae, Jamel, AJ ,David, Braedon, Alyssa, Paul who I have daily chats with and the list goes on. Thank You My Friends. And his group of friends became my group of friends. He even set up a group Facetime call to show they all supported me. Locally I have the 2 George's that help and push me to be a better person and make better decisions.Also my Parent's help with this journey. Thanks Mom and Dad.

So let's get into it and get on to a better you.

3

What to Expect

What To Expect

The first week will be rough. I'm not going to lie to you. It changes your body and you will crave sweets,pizza, soda, and alcohol. BUT you have to refuse it all. It will NOT help you but only hurt you.

I will show you 2 versions of this Diet. One from my Doctor and Health Advisor and the one I adapted for me. It's called the Dartmouth Diet. I personally could not find any information on this But I know it works. I'm Proof and I have helped friends with this.

Just letting you know you will be using the restroom a lot. Lot's of liquids going in and out of you.

This will kick start your metabolism, getting food and protein every 2-2.5 hours. And especially this is all lean clean food and drinks. The pounds melted away. I kept a daily log to weigh myself every morning before breakfast. I had to be true to myself and I built up courage seeing the pounds slipping away.

RESTRICTIONS

If it's not on the list don't eat or drink it. No Bread, Sugar, Soft drinks, Flour, Fried foods NOTHING.

4

Shopping List for Version from Health Advisor

Shopping List from Health Advisor
Oatmeal or Cream of Wheat

Fairlife skim milk

Carnation Breakfast Essentials Light Start or Premier Ready to drink protein drink

Protein Power (if Using Carnation Breakfast Essentials)

Healthy Choice soups

Sugar-free pudding mix

Low fat Greek yogurt

With the items above here's the schedule **then i'll tell you what i changed on my revision.**

5

The Daily Plan Version 1

8 am Breakfast

1 serving of cream of wheat or plain oatmeal prepared with 6-8 oz of Fairlife skim milk

10 am snack

Carnation Breakfast Essentials Light Start mixed with 8 oz of Fairlife skim milk and ½ scoop of protein powder for 8 oz of Fairlife skim milk mixed with 1 scoop of protein powder or 12 oz ready to drink premier protein drink with 30 grams of protein.

12 Noon

1 cup of Healthy choice soup
1 cup of sugar free pudding

2 pm Snack

Same as 10 am snack

4 pm snack

1 serving of low fat Greek yogurt (5.3 oz)

6 pm Dinner
1 cup of Healthy Choice soup

Water drink 8 oz of water or sugar free water 6 times per day 9 am, 11 am 1 pm 3 pm 7 pm

Multivitamin Take 1 multivitamin daily

So Personally This didn't work for me. I'm on the road, I can't cook soup, and need this ready to travel. I also don't like milk, Cream of Wheat or Oatmeal. So here's my shopping list and how I Changed my Diet.

My Shopping List

MY SHOPPING LIST

1. Premier Protein drinks I bought a few cases 2 drinks per day

(I used amazon and Sam's club) I found 7 flavors I liked: Root Beer Float, Bananas and Cream, Cinnamon Rolls, Cookies and Cream, Carmel, Chocolate and Peanut Butter, Cake Batter, Strawberries and cream. These are the ones I liked.

So they have 1 gram of sugar and 30 grams of protein.

2. Sugar free jello and pudding 2 per day

I went to my local supermarket and bought a variety. They have a few flavors of sugar-free puddings and sugar -free jello.

My favorites are sugar-free pudding Vanilla, Chocolate and Dark Chocolate.

As for the sugar-free jello Lime,Strawberry,Orange,Black cherry.

3. **Deli Meats 1 ¼ pound per day**

¼ pound of your favorite deli meats Chicken and Turkey only.

I personally mixed up flavors daily. Chipotle Chicken, cajun Turkey, Buffalo Chicken, BBQ chicken, Fire Roasted Chicken, Salsa Turkey, Pitcraft Turkey,

4 Low fat Greek Yogurt

Check your labels they are NOT ALL THE SAME

I bought OIKOS TRiple ZERO (0 added sugar,0 Artificial sweeteners,0%fat, 15 grams of protein) and only 90 calories. They come in a Black Packaging and have many different flavors.

Here's a few flavors I liked. Banana Creme,Blueberry and Mixed are a few I liked.

5 **Water** 3-4 Bottles per day

This is the key to flushing your body clean.

5.1 **Crystal Light** this helps with the bland flavor of the water. I would use 1 or 2 per day to change up the water flavor.

6 **String Cheese** 3 per week

I used this as a snack 3 times per week to change things up since I don't get much Dairy.

My Daily Plan for 30 days

HERE"S MY DIET SCHEDULE

7 am Premier Protein Drink

9 am-9:30 am Sugar free jello or Pudding

12 noon Deli Meats

2 pm snack sugar free pudding or jello

4-4:30 pm Premier Protein Drink

6-6:30 Greek yogurt

Don't Eat any food 3 Hours before bed. Only Water!!!

I drank black DECaffeinated Tea 3 times a week. NO SUGAR NO CREMERS.

This is the plan I used. This is the Plan that worked for me. As of writing this short book I'm at 331 pounds and FEEL AWESOME. I feel so clean from the fried foods, the soda, the foods that dragged me down.

I personally haven't craved the fried foods, the pizza, the breads and pasta as i did before. It's all about changing your intake for a better you. Make better choices everyday and you will see the difference.

8

Why I had to Change Up My Plan

About Why I had to Change it up

I work a lot, I work long hours and on the road. More about me: I'm a Dj, Sound Engineer. I have worked for Uber and Lyft, DoorDash, Grubhub and even UPS as a seasonal delivery person. So I needed my meals on the go ready for me. I didn't need to be searching for things to eat or drink but to be at my fingertips. As for being a DJ, temptation was at almost every job. From the food served to the guests, the drinks flowing and people offering me food and drinks. I said no thanks. Be strong. It's OK to say no and you must.

Many people didn't know what I was doing. I would take my little cooler into the gigs and into work and it would be good for me. Failure to plan is a Failure for me. It became a routine. I get up at 6:45 am. I weighed myself and put it into my phone. I grab a Premier Protein Drink and drink it as I check my emails overnight. I get dressed and pack my cooler for the day with an ice pack. If I know I'll be out later than 9 pm I have a mini soft cooler to put 2 extra water bottles and a string cheese or pudding in there.

It's all about preparing your day. Make a plan. I set a timer on my phone to go off to make sure I take my next snack or meal. I just went to my local supermarket and bought 6 ¼ pound packages of different deli meats, 12 sugar free puddings and some Crystal light. I keep the Crystal light in my car so it's ready. It is all about changing your habits. When your new routine is a habit it's easy.

9

Exercise

Exercise

Here is another big part. Exercise. Being a Big guy I was or never will be a marathon runner. I walk and keep track of it. Even if you don't walk, start. I started with a walking around my block every morning. Now I do 2 Laps around my neighborhood per day. On Sunday I walked over 13 miles while I was working. Yes 13 miles, I had no clue till we got home. It's a great feat to do. I close my rings everyday on my apple watch and try to do a little more every week. As the weather is getting better go walk at the park, or to the beach and change up the scenery.

Added Exercises you can try

Types of exercise

Cardio, Strength Training, Yoga, Walking, Swimming, Cycling,Weight Lifting, Running,

When creating exercise plans it's very important to find things you like to do and help your goals. Try something new. I tried Hot Yoga, swimming and Bike riding. Gets you out of the house and fresh air vs being in a gym.

Things to keep in mind after the diet try to stay away from processed foods. These foods are often high in salt, sugar and unhealthy fats, and lack essential nutrients needed for a healthy body. As I said a few times, Meal Prep is a key to your health. This will help you make healthy choices and avoid the temptation of Fast Foods and unhealthy snacks. By these simple changes you can improve your energy levels and support your overall fitness and health goals.

Some Benefits and Challenges

Definition of low sugar foods

Low sugar foods are those that contain a minimal amount of added sugars or naturally occurring sugars.These types of foods are often recommended for people looking to reduce levels of diabetes and obesity.

Benefits of low sugar foods.

Lower the risk of developing diabetes. Improved weight management, Better dental Health, Reduced the risk of Heart disease and stroke. Protein Drinks have also gained popularity in recent years. These drinks are often marketed as a convenient and effective way to increase protein intake which is essential for muscle growth and repair. Also a big plus is the protein drinks help you feel FULL. After drinking one I feel full and feel better to move on with my day. Protein drinks are more filling than carbohydrates or fat, so drinking a protein drink can help reduce hunger and prevent overeating. Also protein drinks can help increase muscle mass which can help boost metabolism and burn more calories throughout the day. By adding these protein drinks you get your daily protein levels up without having to have large amounts of dairy and meats.

Here are a few challenges with protein drinks and low sugar foods.

The Cost. Adding these drinks is costly but if you think about going out to lunch nowadays it will cost you $10-$20 per day at a restaurant or sandwich shop. These protein drinks cost me $29.00 for a case of 18 that's $1.66 per drink. That's a bargain.

The biggest thing everywhere you look there are some many companies out there but turn the bottle around and look at the labels. They will be higher in sugars, less protein and more expensive. Or even added sugars or hidden sugars and sweeteners.

But with proper budgeting and planning it is possible to add these drinks into a healthy lifestyle without breaking the bank.

Another challenge of low sugar foods and drinks is the taste. Some people may find the taste of these options not enjoyable as their higher sugar drinks and foods. This can make it difficult to stick to a healthy diet, especially if cravings for sweeter foods persist. IT's all lifestyle change. It took me time to find flavors I liked. I even went to a "health foods store" and they had Girl Scout Cookie flavors. OMG i loved the cookies, but i tried a few flavors, yes they were expensive but only bought a few to satisfy my cravings.

Incorporating low sugar foods and protein drinks into your healthy diet can be a challenge, but it's not impossible. It took me time and lot's of saying no. By understanding the benefits of these options and finding ways to make them enjoyable to eat and drinking know it has improved my Health and my daily routine.

10

Water

Water

Benefits of Water helps with function and mood, as Dehydration can lead to decreased alertness and concentration, as well as irritability and mood swings. Also staying properly hydrated can support healthy skin, as water helps to hydrate skin cells. Drinking water can also help with weight management. It can help reduce hunger and cravings and increase the feeling of being full. Overall water is a crucial part of a healthy lifestyle and should not be overlooked.

Improves overall Health and well being by keeping the body functioning properly.and prevents dehydration. Most adults should consume 8 glasses of water per day. This will help and enhance physical performances to regulate your body temperature. Coffee And alcohol can contribute to dehydration.

Water aids in digestion and helps to flush out toxins from the body in the digestion process. Water also helps boost energy levels and reduces fatigue. Dehydration can lead to feelings of fatigue and low energy levels making it difficult to stay focused and productive throughout the day. By drinking water you can combat these symptoms and boost your energy levels naturally.

Track your water intake daily. They have many apps on the app store to put on your phone to track your water. This is very important to help you reach your goals.Buy a water bottle and keep it with you. If you work in an office you can sip on it all day and fill it up. While at work, at the gym or on the road it will be with you and hydration nearby.

11

After the 30 days

What I Changed after the 30 days

So I have kept the same 2-2 ½ eating schedule everyday. My body is used to it and knows when I'll be eating again. Routine is good.

I went out to eat and had real food. I love Texas roadhouse, pasta rice and more But it's all about limits.

Last week I went to Texas Roadhouse and had a nice healthy salad, a 6oz steak. Yes, I had 2 rolls with their delicious cinnamon butter. But it's all portion control. That was my 1 steak for a month. Yes the bread is bad but again my one stop for the month. OMG I used to have 2 baskets of bread myself. But not anymore. I love it but it's not good for the results I'm looking for. Also I know i'll be back in a month or 2 again. Pace yourself, don't over eat.

Two weeks ago I went out with a friend and had Italian food. A local spot and had a dinner salad with red roasted peppers, homemade oil and vinegar dressing, Baked ziti with meat sauce and a meatball. This was a lunch-sized portion and I couldn't finish it. That's ok i was taking in the greens, peppers and salad as my mains and had the meatball and pasta as the filler. And had my water with lemon as a drink. I was Stuffed and I only had half. My body and stomach has changed to what it needs through the diet. Don't overeat, don't rush your food. Taking your time is a big big thing.

I limit myself to going out 1 time a week. Not going to have the same meal in the same month. Limiting the carbs (pasta,rice,bread) to help me burn it off sooner than later.

12

Conclusion

This was and still is my journey on my weight loss. I hope this Book helps you with your goals. Peace , Love and I hope your Journey goes well.

If you found this Book helpful, I'd be very appreciative if you left a favorable review for the book on Amazon.

Thank You
Derek